New and Emerging Areas in Medicine Series

Quality Improvement and Patient Safety Competencies Across the Learning Continuum

Association of American Medical Colleges

Washington, D.C.

This is a publication of the Association of American Medical Colleges. The AAMC serves and leads the academic medicine community to improve the health of all. aamc.org

Suggested citation: AAMC. *Quality Improvement and Patient Safety Competencies Across the Learning Continuum.* AAMC New and Emerging Areas in Medicine Series. Washington, DC: AAMC; 2019.

ISBN: 978-1-57754-189-9

AAMC

Contents

Association of
American Medical Colleges

Preface

Health care is changing rapidly. New technologies, advances in care delivery, and scientific discoveries are happening at rates that make it challenging for teaching and learning practices across the continuum to keep up. Whether learners are at the beginning of their career or seasoned clinicians, new demands and advances in health care require them to acquire new competencies. The AAMC New and Emerging Areas in Medicine Series is a guide for everyone who develops curricula within the field of medicine and for people learning to practice or continuing their professional development.

Each set of new and emerging competencies, starting with *Quality Improvement and Patient Safety Competencies Across the Learning Continuum*, is developed by leaders from across the medical education and clinical practice communities and is intended to supplement existing competencies (e.g., entrustable professional activities and milestones). The new competencies add depth to selected areas to help guide curricular and professional development, formative performance assessment, cross-continuum collaborations, and, ultimately, improvements in health care services and outcomes. They are not intended for high-stakes assessment or for purposes of accreditation.

Acknowledgments

The AAMC acknowledges the dedication of the talented members of the Expert Working Group, who developed and revised draft competencies and the hundreds of students, residents, faculty, affiliates, patient advocates, and others who reviewed drafts throughout the iterative development process. We thank them for their dedication to advancing patient safety and health care quality through education and collaboration across the continuum.

Expert Working Group

Veronica Catanese, MD, MBA
Senior Director, Accreditation Services, and LCME Secretary
Liaison Committee on Medical Education®

Carol Cronin
Executive Director
Informed Patient Institute

Nancy Davis, PhD
Associate Dean, Continuing Professional Development, and Professor
University of Kansas School of Medicine - Wichita

Linda Headrick, MD, MS
Professor Emerita of Medicine
University of Missouri - Columbia School of Medicine

Eric Holmboe, MD, MACP, FRCP
Senior Vice President, Milestone Development and Evaluation
Accreditation Council for Graduate Medical Education

Kathryn M. Kellogg, MD, MPH
Associate Medical Director
National Center for Human Factors in Healthcare

Rachel Kelz, MD
Professor of Surgery
University of Pennsylvania

Monica Lypson, MD, MHPE
Director of Medical and Dental Education
Department of Veterans Affairs

Kathy McGuinn, MSN, RN, CPHQ
Director of Interprofessional Education and Practice Partnerships
American Association of Colleges of Nursing

Jennifer S. Myers, MD, FHM, FACP
Professor of Clinical Medicine and Assistant Program Director
University of Pennsylvania

Michelle Ogunwole, MD
Chief Resident of Internal Medicine
South Texas Veterans Affairs Hospital

Steve Singer, PhD
Vice President of Education and Outreach
Accreditation Council for Continuing Medical Education

Nathan Spell III, MD
Associate Dean, Education and Professional Development
Emory University

Brian M. Wong, MD, FRCPC
Associate Professor of Medicine
University of Toronto

AAMC Staff
Jennifer Bretsch, MS, CPHQ
Program Management Lead Specialist, Clinical Transformation

Virginia Bush, PMP
Project Manager in Medical Education

Jennifer Faerberg, MHSA
Director of Clinical Transformation

Lisa Howley, PhD, MEd
Senior Director of Strategic Initiatives and Partnerships in Medical Education
QIPS Project Lead

Mallory Lee, MA
Administrative Specialist in Medical Education

Janis Orlowski, MD
Chief Health Care Affairs Officer
Executive Co-Sponsor

Alison Whelan, MD
Chief Medical Education Officer
Executive Co-Sponsor

Series Introduction

Competency-based education (CBE) is a developing approach to health professions education. The AAMC has a long history with CBE and defining the fundamentals for practicing in an increasingly complex health care system. Over the past 20 years, medical education has improved in many ways, including in how outcomes such as competencies are defined and used to guide teaching and learning. To support this kind of positive change, we are offering the New and Emerging Areas in Medicine Series. The series will frame competencies across the undergraduate, graduate, and continuing medical education continuum. This document includes an introduction to CBE, version 1.0 of the first set of competencies, and the context for focusing on quality improvement and patient safety. Details about the development process and a glossary of terms are included as appendixes.

Competency-Based Education

CBE has its roots in primary education and psychology, and its use in medical and other health professions education has grown significantly since the late 1990s. Around that time, the AAMC introduced the Medical School Objectives Project,[1] and the Accreditation Council for Graduate Medical Education (ACGME) and the American Board of Medical Specialties announced six general competency domains for physicians.[2] Before that, schools and programs had been focused more on the processes of curricular or program administration and less on the performance outcomes of learners.

The significant shift from educational processes to outcomes led medical knowledge and patient care domains to expand to interpersonal communication, professionalism, practice-based learning and improvement, and systems-based practice. These six domains are now broadly adopted by other groups within and outside medicine and across the continuum of professional development. They are often a framework for developing a set of competencies, including the current set. A guiding question in developing competencies is, What does a physician, progressing toward attainment of expertise, do, know, and value in relation to the construct in question?

Historical Context of QIPS Focus Area

This series begins by focusing on the constructs of quality improvement and patient safety (QIPS). The QIPS competencies answer the guiding question above and clearly define interdisciplinary competencies for QIPS across the continuum of physician development. This guide will stimulate further integration of QIPS into educational efforts and be a road map for curricular and professional development, performance assessment, and improvement of health care services and outcomes.

Over the past 20 years, in parallel with promising shifts in educational practices, QIPS efforts have also advanced. The year of this publication, 2019, marks the 20th anniversary of the Institute of Medicine's release of *To Err Is Human*.[3] That seminal report started the modern patient safety movement and challenged the medical community to reduce the 44,000 (and perhaps as many as 98,000) deaths and the 1 million patients who were seriously harmed in U.S. hospitals each year through medical errors. Much progress has been made in improving patient safety and continuously enhancing many aspects of care delivery and patients' experience of care. We recognize that medical errors usually result from a complex series of systems-related issues and seldom from the actions of a single provider. Today, awareness of the critical need for lifelong learning to enhance individual skills, team-based communication, and systems improvements is growing.

Despite improvements, patient safety and quality of care still need to be improved across the continuum of physician development — from undergraduate to continuing medical education and practice. Over the past decade, education and training in QIPS have increased significantly at the medical school, residency, and practice levels. However, these efforts have not been developed in a coordinated way across the continuum of medical education. We need to share an understanding and common language for QIPS and value transparency, continuous learning, respectful communication, and engagement of the patient as an active member of the health care team.

In 2009, on the 10th anniversary of *To Err Is Human*, authors of that report said much work remained and the vision they had proposed a decade ago was yet to be realized. Integrating the QIPS competencies across the continuum will bring us much closer to realizing a culture that is "open, transparent, supportive and committed to learning; where doctors, nurses and all health workers treat each other and their patients competently and with respect; where the patient's interest is always paramount; and where patients and families are fully engaged in their care."[4]

Cross-Continuum Competencies: Quality Improvement and Patient Safety

Organization of the Competencies

We developed these competencies over 18 months through an iterative process with extensive stakeholder feedback. (See Appendix A for details.) They are organized into five domains — 1) Patient Safety, 2) Quality Improvement, 3) Health Equity in QIPS, 4) Patients and Families as QIPS Partners, and 5) Teamwork, Collaboration, and Coordination — and three tiers that represent developmental stages in physician development: 1) entry to residency or recent medical school graduate, 2) entry to practice or recent residency graduate, and 3) experienced faculty physician or three to five years post-residency.

Intended Uses

These cross-continuum competencies are intended to help educators design and deliver curricula and related activities and to help learners in their individual QIPS professional development efforts, too. The cross-continuum competencies supplement existing competencies (e.g., entrustable professional activities and milestones) with more detail or depth and guide QIPS curricular and professional development, formative performance assessments, and cross-continuum collaborations and, ultimately, improve health care services and outcomes. They are not intended to be used for high-stakes assessments or accreditation of schools, programs, or institutions. They are for use in:

- Engaging diverse health care professionals in collaborative patient-safety-improvement discussions, including cross-continuum and cross-discipline colleagues.
- Conducting gap analyses of local curricula and training programs.
- Planning individual professional development.
- Developing curricular learning objectives.
- Developing assessment tools.
- Furthering research and scholarship in medical education and quality improvement.
- Guiding the strategic integration of QIPS into the curricula and the clinical learning environment.

Examples of integration tactics are described below (page 4).

Sample Tactics for Improving QIPS Education

- Transform student, resident, and new-physician orientation to focus on patient safety. For example, reprioritize or reframe orientation experiences to educate and reinforce safety protocols and practices.
- Engage patients and families in QIPS efforts by, for example, co-creating curricular activities with patients and family members.
- Use simulation-based education for especially high-risk, infrequent events.
- Include medical educators on sentinel event task forces or committees. Consider common causes that may be addressed through educational interventions and needs or areas for further attention in educational programs.
- Frequently review ACGME Clinical Learning Environment Review (CLER) findings, The Joint Commission (TJC) data, surveys of patient safety culture, and other safety metrics for trends and needs and ask, How can these quality and safety needs inform and be supported by the educational programs and quality improvement efforts of faculty, residents, and students?
- Collaborate closely with colleagues working in quality and safety areas to improve reporting practices, especially of near-miss events.
- Integrate root cause analyses (RCA) into morbidity and mortality (M&M) conferences and daily huddles.
- Share QIPS medical education success stories in governing board meetings, graduate medical education committees (GMECs), and other leadership forums.
- Integrate opportunities to reward safe practices and reporting of near misses or "good catches."

Caveats

Here are some caveats to further clarify the design and use of these competencies:

- Important terms and phrases are defined in the glossary, Appendix B. The competencies are tiered according to level of practice: entry to residency education, entry to independent practice, and experienced faculty physician.
- Depending on local resources and environments, some may consider certain competencies aspirational, and others, as below expectation. We strove to strike a balance between these two extremes. We will apply the lessons learned from the release and use of this version of the report in our constituent communities to the next iteration of the competencies.

- These domains are not mutually exclusive because some competencies may align with more than a single domain. The competencies are organized into the five domains based on the consensus of the Expert Working Group and feedback from hundreds of stakeholders via focus groups and surveys (described below). One notable challenge we faced when constructing the domains was for the "equity" competencies. Although equity is a topic that should be integrated across domains, we called attention to this challenging, important, and relatively unattended area within health care and medical education by including it as the Health Equity in QIPS domain.

- We reviewed several existing and historical competencies, guidelines, and frameworks to prepare the current set of competencies (see Appendix A). To reduce redundancy and increase clarity, we include the relevant harmonized ACGME milestones in this set, noted with the letters "HM" for harmonized milestones and followed by the relevant domain and number. For a complete list of these broader milestones, see Edgar et al.[5]

Feedback on the Competencies

We plan to review and regularly update the competencies based on feedback from the community. We look forward to learning and hearing from you as you use these competencies in creative ways. Please contact QIPS@aamc.org to share feedback, resources, suggestions, and exemplars for teaching and learning.

Resources and Tools

A variety of resources and tools to help people use the competencies are published on the AAMC's MedEdPORTAL®, a peer-reviewed, open-access journal that promotes educational scholarship and dissemination of teaching and assessment resources in the health professions. We welcome submissions for the advancement of medical education!

AAMC

Domain I: Patient Safety

The *Patient Safety* domain is defined as the practices that reduce the occurrence of preventable adverse events and medical errors. The nine competencies in this domain are divided into the subdomains of individual safety practices, safety events, systems safety, and measurement (Table 1).

Table 1. Domain I: Patient Safety

Entering Residency (Recent Medical School Graduate)	**Entering Practice (Recent Residency Graduate)** *All Prior Competencies +*	**Experienced Faculty Physician (3-5 Years Post-Residency)** *All Prior Competencies +*
Individual Safety Practices		
1a. Practices infection-control standard precautions, including but not limited to hand hygiene, use of personal protective equipment, and use and proper disposal of sharps. Uses tools for patient safety including but not limited to "time outs," checklists, medication decision support, and medication reconciliation.	1b. Role models how to perform infection-control practices and ensures the reporting and timely follow-up of injuries, exposures, or both. Follows patient safety protocols and develops processes for their continuous quality improvement (QI). Responds appropriately and in a timely way to decision aids and safety alerts.	1b. Role models infection-control practices and ensures the reporting and timely follow-up of injuries, exposures, or both. Follows patient-safety protocols and develops processes for their continuous QI. Responds appropriately and in a timely way to decision aids and safety alerts.
2a. Practices self-care, including but not limited to seeking help when feeling overwhelmed or in need of support, debriefing with team members after difficult clinical encounters, and knowing how to obtain resources for mental health.	2b. Role models self-care. Recognizes and intervenes when other health care professionals need support.	2c. Identifies and supports the remediation of system factors that contribute to increases in stress and reductions in well-being of health care professionals on the care team.
3a. Accurately and effectively collects key clinical findings needed to inform clinical practice.[1]	3b. Demonstrates clinical reasoning that uses reflection, surveillance, and critical thinking to improve diagnostic performance and mitigate detrimental cognitive bias throughout the clinical encounter.[1]	3c. Role models behaviors that contribute to diagnostic safety that encourages open dialogue and continuous learning from analysis and discussion of excellent diagnostic performance, near misses, and errors.[1]
Safety Events		
4a. Defines and differentiates unsafe conditions, events, and near misses to improve patient safety.	4b. Follows practice-specific protocol for reporting safety events and hazards to improve patient safety.	4c. Role models practice-specific protocol for reporting safety events and hazards to improve patient safety.
5a. Demonstrates knowledge of how to disclose patient safety events.	5b. Discloses patient safety events to patients and families (simulated or actual) (HM-SBP1[2]).	5c. Role models the disclosure of patient safety events.

(continued)

Table 1. Domain I: Patient Safety *(continued)*

Entering Residency (Recent Medical School Graduate)	Entering Practice (Recent Residency Graduate) *All Prior Competencies +*	Experienced Faculty Physician (3-5 Years Post-Residency) *All Prior Competencies +*
6a. Demonstrates knowledge of practice-specific protocol for reporting safety events and hazards to improve patient safety.	6b. Conducts analysis of patient-safety events and offers systems-focused error-prevention strategies (simulated or actual) (HM-SBP1). Manages the immediate harm of an ongoing patient safety event (e.g., gathering information, communicating safety plan).	6b. Conducts analysis of patient-safety events and offers systems-focused error-prevention strategies (simulated or actual) (HM-SBP1). Manages the immediate harm of an ongoing patient safety event (e.g., gathering information, communicating safety plan).
Systems Safety		
7a. Describes common types of human error and limits of human performance.	7b. Promotes behaviors among the health care team that reduce the risk of human error.	7c. As part of an interprofessional team, helps construct system solutions to reduce the risks of human error and of patient safety events.
8a. Describes the role of culture in safety performance. Describes preventable adverse events in the just-culture framework — that is, differentiates among reckless individual contributions to errors, actions, and events that could be remedied with coaching and events that are due to system problems. Identifies system factors and designs that contribute to safe environments of care.	8b. Identifies key elements of and contributes to a culture of patient safety.	8c. Role models behaviors that contribute to a culture of patient safety.
Measurement		
9a. Distinguishes between types of data and tracking methods for targeting patient-safety-improvement efforts.	9b. Participates in a specialty-specific analysis of patient-harm data to target improvement efforts.	9b. Participates in a specialty-specific analysis of patient-harm data to target improvement efforts.

1. Society to Improve Diagnosis in Medicine. Inter-Professional Consensus Curriculum on Diagnosis and Diagnostic Error. https://www.improvediagnosis.org/competency-summary-list/. Accessed Feb. 20, 2019.

2. HM = ACGME Harmonized Milestone; SBP = Systems-Based Practice. For details, see Edgar L, Roberts S, Holmboe E. Milestones 2.0: a step forward. *J Grad Med Ed.* 2018;10(3):367-369. https://doi.org/10.4300/JGME-D-18-00372.1.

Domain II: Quality Improvement

The *Quality Improvement* (QI) domain is defined as the systematic ongoing practices that lead to measurable improvement in health care services and patient outcomes. The 12 competencies in this domain are divided into the subdomains of QI practices, measurement, continuous practice improvement, and high-value care (Table 2).

Table 2. Domain II: Quality Improvement

Entering Residency (Recent Medical School Graduate)	**Entering Practice (Recent Residency Graduate)** *All Prior Competencies +*	**Experienced Faculty Physician (3-5 Years Post-Residency)** *All Prior Competencies +*
QI Practices		
1a. Participates in local system-improvement activities in the context of rotations or learning experiences.	1b. Contributes to local quality-improvement (QI) initiatives in the context of rotations or departmental or institutional efforts.	1c. Role models the skills required to identify, develop, implement, and analyze QI in health care delivery. Creates, implements, and evaluates QI initiatives at the practice, department, service line, institutional, or community level.
2a. Demonstrates knowledge of basic QI methodologies and quality measures (HM-SBP1).	2b. Uses common tools (e.g., flow charts, process maps, fishbone diagrams) to inform QI efforts.	2c. Creates, implements, and evaluates common tools (e.g., flow charts, process maps, fishbone diagrams) to inform QI efforts.
3a. Uses resources to find evidence for health care improvements.	3b. Designs a small test of change to improve some aspect of individual or system performance (using an experimental learning method such as Plan-Do-Study-Act).	3c. Creates, implements, and evaluates small tests of change in daily work (using an experiential learning method such as Plan-Do-Study-Act).
4a. Describes basic principles and approaches for making and sustaining change in QI.	4b. Uses change principles to implement and evaluate tests of change.	4c. Advocates or leads change to enhance systems to improve patient care.
5a. Describes ethical principles that govern QI, including confidentiality of patient information.	5b. Compares and contrasts the ethical principles that govern QI and those for research, including the role of the institutional review board (IRB).	5c. Ensures ethical oversight of QI.
Measurement		
6a. Uses quality measures to identify gaps between local and best practice.	6b. Selects and uses quality measures to understand performance in QI.	6c. Contributes to organizational decision-making in the selection and analysis of quality measures.
7a. Describes strengths, weaknesses, and appropriate uses of measurement and analytic approaches relevant to QI (e.g., run charts, process-control charts).	7b. Interprets QI data displayed in run charts and process-control charts to distinguish significant change from random variation.	7c. Role models the use of measurement and analytic approaches relevant to QI.

(continued)

Table 2. Domain II: Quality Improvement *(continued)*

Entering Residency (Recent Medical School Graduate)	**Entering Practice (Recent Residency Graduate)** *All Prior Competencies +*	**Experienced Faculty Physician (3-5 Years Post-Residency)** *All Prior Competencies +*
Continuous Practice Improvement		
8a. Uses practice data (including report cards, safety events, patient feedback) to inform goals for improvement.	8b. Uses practice data to develop and measure the effectiveness of a learning plan and, when necessary, improves it (HM-PBLI2[1]).	8c. Engages in collaborative learning to continuously improve individual practices and care delivery.
9a. Identifies the factors that contribute to the gap(s) between expectation and actual performance (HM-PBLI2).	9b. Analyzes, reflects on, and institutes behavioral change(s) to narrow the gap(s) between expectations and actual performance (HM-PBLI2).	9c. Role models the value of reflective practice and uses of performance data to inform continuous personal and practice improvements.
High-Value Care		
10a. Recognizes uncoordinated, wasteful, and unnecessary health care delivery.	10b. Manages the interrelated components of the complex health care systems for efficient and effective patient care (HM-SBP3).	10c. Advocates or leads change to enhance systems for high-value, efficient, and effective patient care (HM-SBP3).
11a. Articulates the ethical case for stewarding resources and cost-conscious care, including the potential impact of clinical decisions on whether the patient can afford the cost.	11b. Considers cost when practicing medicine.	11c. Incorporates cost-awareness principles into delivery of complex clinical care.
12a. Recognizes wide variations exist in health care utilization and care delivery patterns across individuals, health systems, and regions that seem to be independent of patients' needs.	12b. Minimizes unnecessary deviation of practice from recommended guidelines or local standards.	12c. Contributes to practice and system-level changes to reduce unnecessary and unwarranted variation.

1. HM = ACGME Harmonized Milestone; PBLI = Practice-Based Learning and Improvement; SBP = Systems-Based Practice. For details, see Edgar L, Roberts S, Holmboe E. Milestones 2.0: a step forward. *J Grad Med Ed.* 2018;10(3):367-369. https://doi.org/10.4300/JGME-D-18-00372.1.

Domain III: Health Equity in QIPS

The *Health Equity in QIPS* domain is defined as the provision of high-quality, safe care to attain the highest level of health for all people. The 10 competencies in this domain are divided into the subdomains of health and health care equity in practice, reporting and using QI data for populations experiencing disparities, physician-level factors contributing to disparities in care, engaging with patients and families to develop QI interventions for populations experiencing health disparities, and physician as advocate for health equity (Table 3).

Table 3. Domain III: Health Equity in QIPS

Entering Residency (Recent Medical School Graduate)	**Entering Practice (Recent Residency Graduate)** *All Prior Competencies +*	**Experienced Faculty Physician (3-5 Years Post-Residency)** *All Prior Competencies +*
Health and Health Care Equity in Practice		
1a. Demonstrates knowledge of population and community health needs and disparities (HM-SBP2[1]). Demonstrates knowledge of local resources available to patients and patient populations with social risk factors.	1b. Participates in changing and adapting practice to provide for the needs of specific populations (HM-SBP2).	1c. Role models the use of and referral to local resources to effectively meet the needs of patients and patient populations with social risk factors.
2a. Collects data about social determinants of health when taking a patient's history.	2b. Describes how social determinants of health affect quality of care for patients experiencing disparities in health care quality.	2c. Tailors care plans around patient-specific social needs.
3a. Explains the importance of the health care system's role in identifying and prioritizing community health needs.	3b. Demonstrates knowledge of the hospital's and health system's efforts to identify and prioritize community health needs.	3c. Explores ways the health system's community health priorities can be used to inform improvement opportunities, teach these concepts, or both.
Reporting and Using QI Data for Populations Experiencing Disparities		
4a. Describes how stratification (e.g., by race/ethnicity, primary language, socioeconomic status, LGBTQ identification) of quality measures can allow for the identification of health care disparities.[2,3]	4b. Explores stratified quality-improvement (QI) data for their patient population and uses this data to identify health care disparities.	4c. Describes how monitoring stratified QI data can help assess the risk of unintended consequences (e.g., widening the disparity gap). Uses stratified QI data to guide and monitor QI interventions.[2]

(continued)

Table 3. Domain III: Health Equity in QIPS *(continued)*

Entering Residency (Recent Medical School Graduate)	**Entering Practice (Recent Residency Graduate)** *All Prior Competencies +*	**Experienced Faculty Physician (3-5 Years Post-Residency)** *All Prior Competencies +*
Physician-Level Factors Contributing to Disparities in Care		
5a. Demonstrates knowledge about the role of explicit and implicit bias in delivery of high-quality care.	5b. Identifies explicit and implicit biases that occur in clinical decision-making.	5c. Role models effective strategies to mitigate explicit and implicit biases that may negatively affect clinical decision-making.
6a. Describes how patients' sociocultural attributes (e.g., values, customs, beliefs) may influence their interactions with the health care system.	6b. Engages with community to explore unique sociocultural attributes (e.g., values, customs, beliefs) that are relevant to the health of populations with health disparities.	6c. Role models how to explore and act upon unique sociocultural attributes of patients.
7a. Identifies the need for and uses appropriate language translation services for relevant patient populations.	7a. Identifies the need for and uses appropriate language translation services for relevant patient populations.	7c. Role models the use of appropriate language translation services for relevant patient populations.
Engaging With Patients and Families to Develop QI Interventions for Populations Experiencing Health Disparities		
8a. Recognizes the importance of engaging and partnering with patient, family, and community in developing effective QI interventions to reduce disparities.	8b. Engages and partners with patient, family, and community in developing effective QI interventions to reduce disparities.	8c. Role models patient, family, community engagement, and partnership in informing strategies to tailor QI interventions.
Physician as Advocate for Health Equity		
9a. Demonstrates knowledge about accessing pathways to physician advocacy.	9b. Participates in local physician-advocacy initiatives.	9c. Leads (or supports) innovations and advocates for populations or communities with health care inequities (HM-SBP2).
10a. Recognizes that systems factors influence health inequities.	10b. Recognizes ways the health system influences health and health care inequities of its local patient population.	10c. Advocates for equity-promoting practice and policy change within their health system and for increased meaningful multisector partnerships to reduce inequities.

1. HM = ACGME Harmonized Milestone; SBP = Systems-Based Practice. For details, see Edgar L, Roberts S, Holmboe E. Milestones 2.0: a step forward. *J Grad Med Ed*. 2018;10 (3):367-369. https://doi.org/10.4300/JGME-D-18-00372.1.

2. Anderson MB, Cohen JJ, Hallock JE, Kassebaum DG, Turnbull J, Whitcomb. *Report I: Learning Objectives for Medical Student Education — Guidelines for Medical Schools.* Washington, DC: AAMC; 1998.

3. Batalden P, Leach D, Swing S, Dreyfus H, Dreyfus S. General competencies and accreditation in graduate medical education: an antidote to overspecification in the education of medical specialists. *Health Aff.* 2002;21:103-111. https://geiselmed.dartmouth.edu/cfm/education/PDF/Article1.pdf. Accessed Aug. 8, 2019.

Domain IV: Patients and Families as QIPS Partners

The *Patients and Families as QIPS Partners* domain is defined as engagements with patients and family that are based on respect, dignity, information sharing, participation, and collaboration in the pursuit of quality improvement and patient safety. The six competencies in this domain are divided into the subdomains of inclusive practice and culturally sensitive shared decision-making (Table 4).

Table 4. Domain IV: Patients and Families as QIPS Partners

Entering Residency (Recent Medical School Graduate)	**Entering Practice (Recent Residency Graduate)** *All Prior Competencies +*	**Experienced Faculty Physician (3-5 Years Post-Residency)** *All Prior Competencies +*
Inclusive Practice		
1a. Identifies opportunities to engage patients and families in improving quality and safety at both the individual and organizational levels.	1b. Participates as a team member with patients and families in efforts to improve quality and safety, including system-level activities.	1c. Intentionally demonstrates for others the inclusion of patients and families in quality-improvement (QI) and patient safety activities at both the individual and organizational levels.
2a. Elicits information from patients and families to identify patient safety hazards or barriers to effective care delivery.	2b. Uses patient- and family-generated data to improve quality and safety.	2c. Role models the use of patient- and family-generated data to improve quality and safety.
3a. Participates in patient safety and QI educational programs that are planned or taught in part by patients or family members.	3b. Partners with patients and families in organized efforts to improve quality and patient safety education.	3c. Role models collaboration with patients and families in planning and teaching practice-based education activities addressing QI and patient safety.
4a. Participates in disclosure of a patient-safety event to patients and families (simulated or actual) (HM-SBP1[1]).	4b. Discloses patient safety events to patients and families (simulated or actual) (HM-SBP1).	4c. Role models the disclosure of patient safety events to patients and families.
Culturally Sensitive Shared Decision-Making		
5a. Demonstrates knowledge of shared decision-making and informed consent. Elicits patient and family goals and preferences about testing and treatment options.	5b. Practices shared decision-making and informed consent with patients and families.	5c. Role models shared decision-making in patient care. Creates and sustains an environment that routinely supports shared decision-making around high-value care.
6a. Identifies common barriers to effective shared decision-making and informed consent and describes effective strategies to address such barriers.	6b. Considers patient preferences and cost effectiveness while promoting patient care that improves outcomes.	6c. Implements organizational strategies to ensure effective shared decision-making and informed consent.

1. HM = ACGME Harmonized Milestone; SBP = Systems-Based Practice. For details, see Edgar L, Roberts S, Holmboe E. Milestones 2.0: a step forward. *J Grad Med Ed*. 2018;10(3):367-369. https://doi.org/10.4300/JGME-D-18-00372.1.

Domain V: Teamwork, Collaboration, and Coordination

The *Teamwork, Collaboration, and Coordination* domain is defined as the knowledge, methods, and skills needed to interact and coordinate effectively in health care settings and to deliver clear information for improved patient outcomes. The seven competencies in this domain are divided into the subdomains of teamwork and collaboration and care coordination (Table 5).

Table 5. Domain V: Teamwork, Collaboration, and Care Coordination

Entering Residency (Recent Medical School Graduate)	Entering Practice (Recent Residency Graduate) *All Prior Competencies +*	Experienced Faculty Physician (3-5 Years Post-Residency) *All Prior Competencies +*
Teamwork and Collaboration		
1a. Describes the role of effective interprofessional and team communication in improving patient safety.	1b. Role models effective and sufficient communications for safe delivery of care.	1c. Role models flexible communication strategies that value input from all health care team members, resolving conflict when needed (HM-ICS2[1]).
2a. Defines "interprofessional collaborative clinical practice." Describes the value that each member of the health care team brings to the delivery of high-quality and safe patient care.	2b. Optimizes the care team. Works as a member of the interprofessional team to address system quality and safety priorities.	2c. Role models interprofessional collaborative clinical practice. Engages in interprofessional continuing education (for the health care team).
3a. Requests a consultation in an organized, succinct, respectful, and timely manner.	3b. Coordinates recommendations from different members of the health care team to optimize patient care (HM-ICS2).	3c. Role models collaborative practice-based learning and improvement.
	4a. Communicates clearly, concisely, in a timely way, and in an organized electronic or written form that includes anticipatory guidance (HM-ICS3).	4b. Role models feedback to improve others' electronic or written communications (HM-ICS3).
Care Coordination		
5a. Gathers and documents a history using sensitive and compassionate methods of inquiry to determine health risk and assets at the point of transition.	5b. Role models effective coordination of patient-centered care in various disciplines and specialties (HM-SBP2).	5c. Role models and advocates for safe and effective transitions of care and handoffs within and across health care delivery systems, including outpatient settings (HM-SBP2).
6a. Articulates the need to facilitate documentation that ensures effective coordination and transition.	6b. Performs handoffs within and across health care delivery systems that incorporate and address as appropriate social determinants of health and the effect on care coordination.	6b. Performs handoffs within and across health care delivery systems that incorporate and address as appropriate social determinants of health and the effect on care coordination.

(continued)

Table 5. Domain V: Teamwork, Collaboration, and Care Coordination *(continued)*

Entering Residency (Recent Medical School Graduate)	Entering Practice (Recent Residency Graduate) *All Prior Competencies +*	Experienced Faculty Physician (3-5 Years Post-Residency) *All Prior Competencies +*
7a. Accurately and appropriately records information in the patient record (HM-ICS3).	7b. Uses an evidence-based approach to patient handovers that includes patient concerns and considerations.	7b. Uses an evidence-based approach to patient handovers that includes patient concerns and considerations.

1. HM = ACGME Harmonized Milestone; ICS = Interpersonal Communication Skills; SBP = Systems-Based Practice.
For details, see Edgar L, Roberts S, Holmboe E. Milestones 2.0: a step forward. *J Grad Med Ed*. 2018;10(3):367-369. https://doi.org/10.4300/JGME-D-18-00372.1

Appendix A. Development Process

There is no single standard approach to the development of competencies, but there are some preferred steps:

1. Define the scope of the competencies or the construct.
2. Engage diverse stakeholders and collect data to understand the nature of the construct. How do high performers perform? How do those who achieve positive results behave in practice? Gather data through literature reviews, focus groups, and electronic surveys of subject matter experts.
3. Draft the competencies.
4. Have reactor panels of subject matter experts, patients, frontline clinicians, and educators review the competencies.
5. Importantly, review and update competencies periodically to keep pace with changes in clinical and educational practices.

We followed those steps to develop the QIPS competencies and describe the methods we used below.

In 2017, the AAMC began developing QIPS competencies across the continuum of physician development. This collaboration was informed by our constituents in medical education and clinical affairs who, despite advances in areas of QIPS education, continue to struggle to effectively demonstrate strong, broad QIPS outcomes. A diverse working group (listed on page v) of educators, clinicians, advocates, and accreditation leaders was formed in fall 2017 with the charge of developing consensus on interdisciplinary tiered competencies for QIPS, building from and informed by existing work. This diverse group initially reviewed the literature and existing educational competencies on QIPS education, including the following:

- AAMC CoreEPA Toolkit 13.
- AAMC Te4Q 2015 draft competencies.
- ACGME CLER Pathways Report.
- Quality and Safety Education for Nurses (QSEN) Competencies.
- CanMEDS 2015 Framework.
- National Association for Healthcare Quality (NAHQ) Certified Professional in Healthcare Quality (CPHQ) Examination Blueprint.
- Institute for Healthcare Improvement (IHI) Open School Course Learning Objectives.[6-11]

This existing work informed the development of an initial list of domains and, eventually, draft competencies for the following five domains: Patient Safety; Quality Improvement; Patients and Families as QIPS Partners; Teamwork, Collaboration, and Coordination; and Health Equity in QIPS.

Once the domains and competencies were drafted, we took multiple approaches to collecting stakeholder feedback. We collected early feedback at nine focus groups of constituents from across the country at several AAMC meetings and at an Association of State and Territorial Health Officials meeting. The AAMC affiliate group meetings included all four regions of the Group on Educational Affairs (Northeast, South, West, and Central), the Group on Resident Affairs, and the Health Equity Meeting of the Research on Care Community Health Equity, as well as the AAMC Integrating Quality Conference.

In addition to surveying via focus groups, we used a modified Delphi method to further refine the competencies and increase stakeholder input. This included developing a questionnaire of standard items (see the Survey Questions box on page 17), conducting iterative email rounds with that questionnaire and focus groups, collecting individual or group feedback between rounds, and summarizing the findings. An electronic questionnaire inviting feedback about the initial domains and competencies was initially distributed to 185 stakeholders in May 2018. The stakeholders who received that questionnaire included people engaged in health professions education, quality improvement, patient safety, faculty development, public health, hospital administration, and clinical services. In addition to gathering feedback from those stakeholders and the panel of reactors, we invited more than 60 organizations to review and refine the competencies. We used the feedback from the first iteration to revise the domains and the competencies and made multiple changes to the competencies across the three tiers and within all domains.

The second questionnaire was sent in August 2018 to 217 stakeholders and included the same questions as the first version but a revised set of domains and competencies.

The response rates for the first and second surveys were 31% and 30%, respectively. We analyzed the mixed-methods data from the two surveys and further revised the competencies. Three domains were the same in both iterations: Patient Safety, Quality Improvement, and Patients and Families as Partners in QIPS. Responses to 80% of the questions in the second questionnaire were as or more favorable than responses to the first questionnaire. Overall, there was a slightly more favorable response to the second questionnaire, with 90% (compared with 87%) indicating the competencies "will be helpful to them as they educate students, residents and/or physician faculty." We then shared the draft of the QIPS domains and competencies again with the Expert Working Group for further refinement. The final version 1.0 of the QIPS competencies is on pages 6-14. We defined *consensus* as middle ground, between total assent and total disagreement, and the working group reached consensus on the final version 1.0 after three formal drafts.

Survey Questions About Draft Domains and Competencies

Respondents, including focus group members and reactor panelists, reviewed the draft domains and related competencies and answered the following five standard questions about each domain:

1. **Importance** - Does this set of draft competencies represent abilities that are important to high quality, safe care? Response Options: 1 - Not At All, 3 - Unsure, 5 - Yes, Definitely. Please describe your response:

2. **Tier** - Does this set of draft competencies reflect observable abilities at the appropriate level for a new resident, new physician faculty, or experienced physician faculty? Response Options: 1 - Not At All, 3 - Unsure, 5 - Yes, Definitely. Please describe your response:

3. **Comprehensive** - Does this set of draft competencies reflect the full domain or are there specific abilities that are missing? Response Options: 1 - Not At All, 3 - Unsure, 5 - Yes, Definitely. Please describe your response:

4. **Granularity** - Does the language reflect an optimal consistent level of granularity? Response Options: 1 - Too Vague, 2 - Just Right! 3 - Too Specific, 4 - Not Sure. Please describe your response:

5. **General feedback on this set of competencies:**

At the end of the questionnaire, respondents were asked to consider the full set of draft competencies in the five QIPS domains and answer four questions:

1. **What, if anything, is missing?** (open-ended)

2. **Do the five domains listed appropriately represent the breadth of QIPS?** Please explain:

3. **Do these draft competencies represent the depth of QIPS?** Please explain:

4. **Do you believe these competencies will be helpful to your or your colleagues as they educate students, residents, and/or physician faculty?** Please explain:

Appendix B. Glossary

anticipatory guidance: "Information about normal expectations of an age group (or of a disease) to provide support for coping with problems before they arise. It is a component of many health care encounters, e.g., well-child checkups in infancy."[13]

care plan: "A written, personalised care plan, which, under the single-assessment process, details a patient's integrated health and social care needs."[13]

competency-based medical education: "An outcomes-based approach to the design, implementation, assessment, and evaluation of medical education programs, using an organizing framework of competencies."[14]

consensus: "Middle ground, between total assent and total disagreement."[1]

experienced faculty physician: A medical doctor who has completed medical school (MD or DO) and residency, has completed at least three years of independent practice, and teaches or supervises learners, either paid or volunteer, full- or part-time.

explicit bias: "The traditional conceptualization of bias. With explicit bias, individuals are aware of their prejudices and attitudes toward certain groups. Positive or negative preferences for a particular group are conscious."[16]

handoff or handover: "The passing of the care of one or more patients to the doctors and nurses working on the next shift, by informing them of tests ordered, management issues and evolving or resolving problems."[13]

health equity in QIPS: The provision of high-quality, safe care to attain the highest level of health for all people.

high-value care: "The best care for the patient, with the optimal result for the circumstances, delivered at the right price."[17]

implicit bias: "Also known as unconscious bias, refers to attitudes or stereotypes that are outside our awareness but nonetheless affect our understanding, our interactions, and our decisions."[18]

informed consent: "Permission obtained from a patient to perform a specific test or procedure. Informed consent is required before most invasive procedures are performed and before a patient is admitted to a research study."[19]

just culture: "A culture in which frontline personnel feel comfortable disclosing medical errors — including their own — while maintaining professional accountability. A just culture recognizes that competent professionals make mistakes."[20]

medical error: "An act of commission (doing something wrong) or omission (failing to do to right thing) that leads to an undesirable outcome or significant potential for such an outcome."[20]

near miss: "An event or situation that did not produce patient injury, but only because of chance. This good fortune might reflect robustness of the patient or a fortuitous, timely intervention."[20]

patient safety: The practices that reduce the occurrence of preventable adverse events and medical errors.

patient safety event or adverse event: "An injury caused by medical care."[20]

patients and families as QIPS partners: Engagements with patients and families based on respect, dignity, information sharing, participation, and collaboration in the pursuit of quality improvement and patient safety.

Plan-Do-Study-Act (PDSA): "The cycle of activities advocated for achieving process or system improvement. The components of the cycle include: Plan, Do, Study and Act."[20]

quality improvement: The systematic ongoing practices that lead to measurable improvement in health care services and patient outcomes.

role model: "One who serves as an example for others by demonstrating the behavior associated with a particular social position or profession."[19]

run chart: "A type of statistical process-control or quality-control graph in which some observation is plotted over time to see if there are 'runs' of points above or below a center line, usually representing the average or median. In addition to the number of runs, the length of the runs conveys important information. If a nonrandom change for the better, or shift, occurs, it suggests that an intervention has succeeded."[20]

shared decision-making: "A process in which clinicians and patients work together to make decisions and select tests, treatments, and care plans based on clinical evidence that balances risks and expected outcomes with patient preferences and values."[21]

social risk factors: "A set of constructs that capture the key ways in which social processes and social relationships could influence key health-related outcomes. The five domains of social risk factors are socioeconomic position (SEP); race, ethnicity, and cultural context; gender; social relationships; and residential and community context."[22]

teamwork, collaboration, and coordination: The knowledge, methods, and skills needed to interact and coordinate effectively in health care settings and to deliver clear information for improved patient outcomes.

References

1. Anderson MB, Cohen JJ, Hallock JE, Kassebaum DG, Turnbull J, Whitcomb. *Report I: Learning Objectives for Medical Student Education — Guidelines for Medical Schools*. Washington, DC: AAMC; 1998.

2. Batalden P, Leach D, Swing S, Dreyfus H, Dreyfus S. General competencies and accreditation in graduate medical education: an antidote to overspecification in the education of medical specialists. *Health Aff*. 2002;21:103-111. https://geiselmed.dartmouth.edu/cfm/education/PDF/Article1.pdf. Accessed Aug. 8, 2019.

3. Institute of Medicine Committee on Quality of Health Care in America; Kohn LT, Corrigan JM, Donaldson MS, eds. *To Err Is Human: Building a Safer Health System*. Washington, DC: National Academy Press; 2000.

4. Leape L, Berwick D, Clancy C, et al. Transforming healthcare: a safety imperative. *BMJ Qual Saf*. 2009;18:424-428.

5. Laura E, Roberts S, Holmboe E. Milestones 2.0: A step forward. *J Grad Med Educ*. 2018;10(3):367-369.

6. Obeso V, Brown D, Aiyer M, et al., eds. *Core EPAs for Entering Residency Pilot Program. Toolkits for the 13 Core Entrustable Professional Activities for Entering Residency*. Washington, DC: AAMC; 2017. https://www.aamc.org/initiatives/coreepas/publicationsandpresentations/. Accessed Aug. 8, 2019.

7. AAMC Teaching for Quality Expert Panel. *Integrating Quality Improvement and Patient Safety Across the Continuum of Medical Education*. Washington, DC: AAMC; 2013. https://www.aamc.org/initiatives/meded/494232/te4qreport.html. Accessed Aug. 8, 2019.

8. ACGME Clinical Learning Environment Review (CLER). National report of findings. 2018. *J Grad Med Educ*. 2018;10(4 Suppl):1-80. https://www.jgme.org/toc/jgme/10/4s. Accessed Aug. 8, 2019.

9. Cronenwett L, Sherwood G, Gelmon S. Improving quality and safety education: the QSEN learning collaborative. *Nurs Outlook*. 2009;57:304-312.

10. Frank JR, Snell L, Sherbino J, eds. *CanMEDS 2015 Physician Competency Framework*. Ottawa: Royal College of Physicians and Surgeons of Canada; 2015.

11. National Association for Healthcare Quality. CPHQ Exam Blueprint Outline. https://nahq.org/certification/content-outline. Accessed Aug. 8, 2019.

12. Institute for Healthcare Improvement. Open School Course. http://www.ihi.org/education/ihiopenschool/Pages/default.aspx. Accessed Aug. 8, 2019.

13. Segen JC. *The Dictionary of Modern Medicine*. Park Ridge, NJ: Parthenon Publishing Group;1992.

14. Frank JR, Snell LS, Cate OT, et al. Competency-based medical education: theory to practice. *Med Teach*. 2010;32(8):638-645.

15. WebFinance Inc. BusinessDictionary.com. http://www.businessdictionary.com/definition/consensus.html. Accessed Aug. 13, 2019.

16. U.S. Department of Justice. *Understanding Bias: A Resource Guide*. Washington, DC: U.S. Department of Justice. 2015. https://www.justice.gov/crs/file/836431/download. Accessed Aug. 8, 2019.

17. Committee on the Learning Health Care System in America, Institute of Medicine; Smith M, Saunders R, Stuckhardt L, et al., eds. *Best Care at Lower Cost: The Path to Continuously Learning Health Care in America*. Washington, DC: National Academies Press; 2013.

18. AAMC. *Unconscious Bias in Academic Medicine: How the Prejudices We Don't Know We Have Affect Medical Education, Medical Careers, and Patient Health.* Washington, DC: AAMC; 2017.

19. Myers T, ed. *Mosby's Medical Dictionary.* 8th ed. St. Louis, MO: Mosby Elsevier; 2009.

20. Agency for Healthcare Research Quality, U.S. Department of Health and Human Services. Patient Safety Network (AHRQ PSNet). https://psnet.ahrq.gov/glossary. Accessed Aug. 8, 2019.

21. National Learning Consortium, HealthIT.gov. Shared Decision Making Fact Sheet. https://www.healthit.gov/sites/default/files/nlc_shared_decision_making_fact_sheet.pdf. Accessed Aug. 8, 2019.

22. National Academies of Sciences, Engineering, and Medicine. *Accounting for Social Risk Factors in Medicare Payment: Identifying Social Risk Factors*. Washington, DC: National Academies Press; 2016.

Made in the USA
Monee, IL
05 November 2026

67379805R00019